How to Grow Psilocybin Mushrooms: The Complete Beginners Guide to Indoor Cultivation

Written By Carl E Miller
Published By Mushroom Insider

Chapter 1: Gathering essential items

Chapter 2: Grow room set-up

Chapter 3: Inoculation, Incubation and Colonization

Chapter 4: Fruiting

Chapter 5: Identifying, Picking, Drying Finished Product and Other Tricks and Techniques Including Grain to Grain Transfer

Introduction:

In order to grow mushrooms correctly, patience and cleanliness is definitely the most important practice. There are numerous websites that offer everything that will be needed to complete this process. In some cases you will need to order the mushroom spores from one site, and the growing materials from a separate site.

I will cover multiple ways to approach each step, including results from my own personal experiences using these techniques. I will take you through every single step, and by the time you have completed this book you will no longer be an amateur grower, I guarantee it. After more than a decade of growing mushrooms, I've condensed everything that I've learned into a simple guide that literally anyone can easily understand.

If you follow this guide closely, it should be essentially error proof. With that being said, always be prepared to handle any sort of contamination immediately, before it spreads and becomes uncontrollable. If at any time during the growing process you suspect mold to be on your substrate, always be safe and throw it away. Mycelium growth is pure white and you should never, under any circumstances, see any other color growth on your substrate. NEVER!

Psilocybin mushrooms have been used medicinally for centuries, and now in one easy read, you can grow them just as powerful as the best professional grower. The start-up cost for growing mushrooms is significantly cheaper than most of the alternatives, such as marijuana which can become quite expensive with the lights (and cost of using those lights).

Mushrooms don't use much light, mainly just to direct them which way to grow. Although it's a rather cheap experiment, it can definitely become a time-consuming process that can be frustrating until it's picking time, then your patience is rewarded.

The more time you put in, the better your result will be. Don't get frustrated easily because this is a learning process and some mushroom strains do better in certain environments than others, so always look for resilient strains that do well in the substrate of your choice.

For a rough estimation, if you want a good turnout, then you will be spending several hours building and cleaning your room just to get you started. Inoculating your jars (injecting spores) will take some time as well, especially to make sure everything is completely sterile.

After inoculation you will have a few weeks waiting around break, then during the fruiting stages you will need to dedicate an hour or two worth of time for fanning, misting and temperature check-ins every day. Do not slack on any steps, or your yield will suffer greatly.

Chapter 1: Gathering Essential Items

All of the items that will be posted below are readily available and can be found at reputable online stores such as MidwestGrowKits.com (which I highly recommend), and Spores101.com (which I also highly recommend). These two stores will cover your spores and your Mushrooms growing medium needs.

Spores (Basidiospore) are basically the mushroom seed and you can purchase this in multiple ways including in a syringe, diluted with water (this is the recommended method that will be covered below), a spore print and live culture. The spore print and live culture methods are far trickier to master, and are therefore only recommended for seasoned growers.

The spores that I've had the most success with are Golden Teacher, Albino and the B+ strains which grow very strong and fast. The growing medium is just as important as the spores, and comes in many varieties including straw, grain, sawdust, manure and worm castings, with each having their own pros and cons.

Now that we've established what spores and a growing medium are, let's continue to the choices of packaging that the medium will arrive in. I've used two different types personally, jars and bags, with again both having their pros and cons which I will break down.

First you have the 8oz (or any size you choose) ultimate substrate jars, which typically contains brown rice flour with vermiculite, mineral water, Liquid worm castings and Bee pollen, or the multi grain jars. These are particularly great for first-time growers or anyone who wants a fast turnaround. The mushroom spawn bags are slightly more complicated, but the reward can potentially be much higher.

The mushroom spawn bags are much larger than the 8oz or 12oz jars, the spawn bags vary in weight, usually 2lbs, 3lbs, 5lbs, 10lbs and 20lbs with the larger obviously taking way longer to colonize (mycelium growth). Spawn bags, as well as some of the modern jars have self healing injection ports (which basically means after injecting with a syringe the hole that is left behind self-heals, preventing future contamination).

The multigrain bags and jars are always a great choice, these are available at MidwestGrowKits.com. Now that we've covered the mushroom jars and spawn bag aspect, next we need a 12 gallon bag of perlite, aluminum foil and a small spray water bottle. Another very important item that will be needed is the UV magic wand sanitizing light, shop around a little for the best price. You will also need a humidifier if you really want the best results.

This light will be essential for the inoculation (syringe injection) process. Now we will need a <u>Clear</u> see-through Rubbermaid container (preferably a 30+ gallon, Roughneck Rubbermaid with clear sides and a clear lid). You will now need to get a 4inch by 2ft PVC pipe (if you plan on using a humidifier).

Next you will need to order plenty of sanitizer, sanitizer wipes, disinfectant spray(some people prefer bleach), some sort of light, a temperature gauge, a few ounces of vermiculite, box of 1 gallon (or any size large enough to hold the medium) ziplock bags, and have a sharp knife or icepick handy. A 60 watt light is sufficient, nothing too powerful, I prefer a small light that can stick to the ceiling, especially one that has a blue tint.

Now you will need five final items and we can proceed to the next chapter. Gorilla tape, a 6x8 tarp (from Home Depot or Walmart), an air conditioner filter, a 40 inch open nylon zipper and an oil-filled radiator space heater (if your house isn't at an optimal temperature, then this exact heater is necessary).

Let's double check before we carry on....

- Spore syringe
- Grow medium
- 2 Rubbermaid container
- Perlite
- Vermiculite
- Aluminum foil
- Sanitizer wipes
- Disinfectant spray
- Air conditioner filter
- Nylon zipper
- UV magic wand light
- Light
- Oil-filled space heater
- Tarp
- Temp gauge
- Ziplock bags
- Humidifier

- 4inch by 2ft PVC pipe

Chapter 2: Grow Room Set-up

Now this part will differ greatly depending on your approach, and your room of choice that you will be growing in. I prefer a smaller room, especially for beginners, so a walk-in closet works the best in my experience. Something like 6ft long, 3ft wide and 8ft high is the average dimensions of a walk-in closet.

If you choose to create a different style room that is just fine, if you're going to use the closet then we will start with the door. First remove the door if one is present, second we will use the recently bought 6x8ft tarp as our temporary door. Next you will create an entrance by making a makeshift door, using the aforementioned nylon zipper. In order to do this you can look up a DIY video available for free on YouTube, but there's really not much to it.

Next you will cut a square that your air conditioner filter will rest in near the top half of the door, using gorilla tape to seal it shut. This will protect your grow room from unwanted contaminants, which have the potential to shatter your growing dreams. With your new filter/window your room can now breathe safely, if done correct.

Now that you have your door built, filter/window created and sealed, next we will turn our clear Rubbermaid container into an incubation/fruiting chamber. In the near future we will be layering around 4-6 inches of damp perlite in the bottom of the container, so for now take a sharp knife or a drill and make several very small holes down both sides of the container, on the lower 4-6 inch area so the future perlite can breathe.

After you have made small punctures on both lower sides of the container, do the exact same on the upper half of the container, but not as high, a little above the middle will work. After completion you should have about two dozen small holes spread out evenly in the areas explained above, this is called a shotgun chamber fruiting chamber, which you can make unique to your own personal preferences.

With your other Rubbermaid container, you will place the humidifier in and cut a 4inch hole in both containers, in order to run the PVC pipe from one to the other. This is how you will get your humidity that is necessary for good growth, into the grow chamber without flooding the cakes with too much water.

Now we will use the 12 gallon bag of perlite to layer the bottom of the container with. This has covered everything needed for your grow room and incubation/fruiting chamber to be complete. At this point you can begin cleaning everything with the sanitizer wipes and disinfectant spray. This part is very important so truly clean every inch of your grow room.

If you have shelves in your closet this would be great for storing the substrate jars for the Inoculation, incubation and colonization process. In fact you can cover the shelves so no light enters, and use the closet for both colonization and incubation. I have done this with success because the more that you can limit to one room, the better.

You can have your shotgun chamber (Rubbermaid container with holes drilled) on the ground, or on top of another container to keep the temperature up if needed, and being off the ground reduces chances of contamination. Then you can store your jars/bags that are colonizing in the shelves so they can be stored in the dark, the temperature shouldn't be an issue.

Everytime you enter the room (either to check-up on the colonization process or to fan/mist your cakes) make sure you and your clothes are completely fresh and clean. I will mention this several times because believe me, it's extremely important. If your grow fails, 99% of the time it will be because of contamination in one way or another.

Everyone who grows for long enough will experience contamination, but if caught early on you can stop the spread. This is why being as clean as possible, along with the custom (air-conditioner filter window) to keep dust particles out, because one tiny little dust particle can and will completely ruin a grow if you're not careful.

Your operation is most at risk early on, during the colonization period. This is due to the fact that once the cake is colonized, there is no longer usable substrate for the mold to feast on. This doesn't mean that your mycelium can't develop mold, it definitely can. If your growing environment isn't correct you will develop pink, green and even brown growths which will need to be tossed.

Chapter 3: Inoculation, Incubation and Colonization

Now at this stage some people use the glove box method, which I personally do not use. If you would like to search that method for this part you obviously can, if not just be certain your grow room, clothes and body are perfectly clean. Keep in mind, one single dust particle could make contact with your substrate, resulting in contamination.

After everything is clean you can now bring in your jars/bags and spores into the grow room. Now the site you bought your spores from should have instructed you how many cc's to inject, for jars (0.3 cc's) and bags (0.6cc's) are usually the recommendation. Make sure you take a sanitizer wipe to the syringe, let it dry, and have the magic wand scanning about 1ft above when you inject the spore syringe into the inoculation point(s) of the jars/bags, make sure to distribute the spores evenly.

In some cases this can be slightly difficult so perhaps rig something together to hold the UV light, that way the magic wand is scanning the syringe during inoculation (avoid contact with skin or eyes). This is a precautionary step after you have already sanitized the syringe and cleaned yourself and the room perfectly.

After inoculation, you will want to store your jars/bags in a dark room at a temperature range preferably between 65 and 70 degrees. Over the next few weeks the colonization will occur, this is the incubation and colonization process, you can check in maybe once a week to monitor. Look for healthy mycelium growth (white growth) on the medium substrate. Make sure you're very clean every time you enter the room. You will know when the colonization is complete, when your entire substrate has been taken over with mycelium growth. If you're using bags this step will take longer and in some cases you can lightly shake the bag to encourage growth.

After it appears your jars/bags have been fully colonized, wait a few extra days to be certain. Always throw away anything that appears to be mold (black, odd fluffy white mold which is different from mycelium, pink, green or black). Waiting a little longer is always better than not long enough, if you wait too long mushrooms will grow from within the bag or jar, but no harm done. If you don't wait long enough, your substrate may not be fully colonized and could be at potential risk for contamination.

Your substrate will visibly shrink some after it is fully colonized, making it easy to simply flip the jar upside down and a light tap should free the cake, as for the bags again they take a bit longer, make sure they are fully colonized, not just colonized on the outside. If you're using both jars and bags, then your bags will likely need to be separated at this point, in order to finish colonizing, then you can reintroduce all of the cakes again.

There is no issue with using cakes from a jar or bag, as long as they're fully colonized. The only difference is if the jars you chose are anything other than grain, then you won't be able to attempt the grain-to-grain transfer.

Chapter 4: Fruiting

After the jars/bags are completely ready you will fill the ziplock bags with cold water, then dunk the cakes (colonized substrate medium) into the bags. Be sure the substrate is fully submerged, then place the bags in a cool room or a refrigerator for anywhere from 8-16 hrs. With experience you will begin to determine the time that works best for you, but never push past 16hrs or they will drown.

In this process you can also learn a lot with a digital scale, by weighing the cakes before and after dunking to observe how much water they're holding. Later on when you become experienced you will be able to judge future yields by the weight of the cakes.

While you wait for your cakes to absorb water, you can add the perlite layer to the bottom of your Rubbermaid container. Before pouring the perlite, add water in order for the perlite to work properly. Don't soak the perlite too much, but make sure it's all nice and damp. Do not leave any puddles of water.

Now you can take your aluminum foil and cut them into square pieces, large enough for your cakes to rest on. Just make the squares large enough, that when the cake sits on the foil only a little bit of the foil is visible, around the entire cake. This helps from your mushrooms growing downward instead of up, and so the perlite doesn't damage your cake.

The 60 watt (or small blue light) that you chose will also encourage upward growth, so be sure the light is directly above the container. Also that is why the clear lid was so important, do not use a powerful light and so not put a light too close to the cakes, besides the UV light which will not harm mycelium.

Now your room and your chamber is completely ready, so after your cakes have finished dunking you will need the vermiculite. Take the cakes that have fully absorbed water, dunk the cakes in a full layer of vermiculite, where the entire cake is layered lightly. The vermiculite will help the cake hold water, and fight off contaminants.

After you have dunked your cakes in water, rolled them in vermiculite, you will now place them on the prepared square pieces of aluminum foil that should be sitting on the layer of vermiculite in your chamber. Next you will take your spray bottle and mist the sides and lid of your container, along with lightly misting the cakes. Add a little extra vermiculite on the top of the cake, to hold more water when you mist.

Now the ideal fruiting temperature for your room would be 60 degrees. If you have a hard time naturally keeping your room above 55 degrees, then you will need to bring in your oil-filled space heater. At this point you should have one clear container filled with a layer of perlite, aluminum squares on top of perlite, and cakes layered in damp vermiculite on top of squares. Your sides and lid should be well misted. Your other container should be connected by way of PVC pipe, and should also be hosting the humidifier that you will only use as needed. Do not just leave the humidifier constantly on, or you will flood cakes. Only turn the humidifier on for an hour or so a day and change the air filter monthly, or you will have unclean air exchange which will be devastating.

Now the only thing left to do while you wait for your mushrooms to appear is mist fanning. This can be done with your spray bottle and the container's lid, which you will remove and slightly fan the cakes several times a day for fresh air exchange, which is incredibly important. As well mist everytime before you fan, lightly a few feet above the cakes.

Keep in mind the more you fan, the heavier your fruits will be. Again fanning is INCREDIBLY important to both healthy growth and not having a contamination issue from stale air. Always fan after misting, don't allow water to accumulate too much on your cakes, creating rot.

I have also found that using a small light that has a blue tint works very well, placing it right on the top of the container and only leaving it on for an hour or two a day. Again that's why the clear lid is very important, the light directs the mushrooms where to grow, if the light comes in from the sides, the mushrooms will grow sideways.

Chapter 5: Identifying, Picking, Drying Finished Product and Other Tricks and Techniques Including Grain to Grain Transfer

Now when identifying the Mushrooms you will want to look closely for any oddities that may include molds or any kind of rotting. If they seem healthy you will want to wait until the cap seems as it's just about to break from the stem, this is the process in nature in which the spores are released. When you pick the mushrooms, you will want to pinch gently as close to the substrate base as possible, and slightly twist and pull at the same time.

You will want to wait until the majority of the mushrooms on the cake are ready, and pick them all at once. After picking the mushrooms you will notice little dents or craters left behind, these areas will be more susceptible to contamination. You can combat this by dunking the cakes again, after lightly scraping off the old vermiculite. This is also necessary to regain the water weight to produce more mushrooms, and then you can recoat them in vermiculite, for protection.

After you have picked your mushrooms you can begin drying them. What I enjoy doing is slicing the mushrooms in half, which will help the dry faster and you can see the drug present. By this I mean the visible color blue which can also be seen on the cakes (appears as bruising, especially after dunking or handling too rough).

If your mushrooms are strong, then you will know after you slice into one, because it will be as dark blue as a